Recommended Standards for Delivering High-Quality Care to Veterans with Invisible Wounds

CARRIE M. FARMER, SIERRA SMUCKER, NATALIE ERNECOFF, HAMAD AL-IBRAHIM

Sponsored by the George W. Bush Institute, the Bob Woodruff Foundation, and Wounded Warrior Project

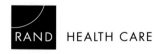

HEALTH CARE

For more information on this publication, visit **www.rand.org/t/RRA1728-1**.

About RAND

The RAND Corporation is a research organization that develops solutions to public policy challenges to help make communities throughout the world safer and more secure, healthier and more prosperous. RAND is nonprofit, nonpartisan, and committed to the public interest. To learn more about RAND, visit www.rand.org.

Research Integrity

Our mission to help improve policy and decisionmaking through research and analysis is enabled through our core values of quality and objectivity and our unwavering commitment to the highest level of integrity and ethical behavior. To help ensure our research and analysis are rigorous, objective, and nonpartisan, we subject our research publications to a robust and exacting quality-assurance process; avoid both the appearance and reality of financial and other conflicts of interest through staff training, project screening, and a policy of mandatory disclosure; and pursue transparency in our research engagements through our commitment to the open publication of our research findings and recommendations, disclosure of the source of funding of published research, and policies to ensure intellectual independence. For more information, visit www.rand.org/about/principles.

RAND's publications do not necessarily reflect the opinions of its research clients and sponsors.

Published by the RAND Corporation, Santa Monica, Calif.
© 2022 RAND Corporation
RAND® is a registered trademark.

Library of Congress Control Number: 2022907058
ISBN: 978-1-9774-0868-6

Cover: photo by Grant Miller for the George W. Bush Presidential Center

About This Report

The Veteran Wellness Alliance, an initiative of the George W. Bush Institute, aims to connect post-9/11 veterans with peer networks and high-quality care for the invisible wounds of war, including posttraumatic stress disorder (PTSD), depression, substance use disorders, and mild traumatic brain injury (TBI). To further its mission, the Veteran Wellness Alliance asked the RAND Corporation to develop a definition of high-quality care for these conditions. A proposed definition of high-quality care for PTSD and TBI was described in a previous report (Farmer and Dong, 2020). In this report, we expand the definition to include additional types of invisible wounds (depression and substance use) and recommend a set of standards for the delivery of high-quality care for these conditions. We also provide considerations for implementing and disseminating these standards as a first step to improve access to high-quality care for veterans with invisible wounds.

This research was funded by the George W. Bush Institute, the Bob Woodruff Foundation, and Wounded Warrior Project and carried out within the Quality Measurement and Improvement Program in RAND Health Care.

RAND Health Care, a division of the RAND Corporation, promotes healthier societies by improving health care systems in the United States and other countries. We do this by providing health care decisionmakers, practitioners, and consumers with actionable, rigorous, objective evidence to support their most complex decisions. For more information, see www.rand.org/health-care, or contact

RAND Health Care Communications
1776 Main Street
P.O. Box 2138
Santa Monica, CA 90407-2138
(310) 393-0411, ext. 7775
RAND_Health-Care@rand.org

Acknowledgments

The authors would like to thank Kacie Kelly, Matt Amidon, Jen Silva, Margaret Harrell, and the Veteran Wellness Alliance clinical and peer-network partners for their help with and support of this report. They would like to acknowledge funding support from the George W. Bush Institute, the Bob Woodruff Foundation, and Wounded Warrior Project. Finally, they thank Paula Schnurr and RAND colleagues Kimberly Hepner, Paul Koegel, and Jeanne Ringel for their reviews of this work, as well as Aaron Lang and Rosa Maria Torres from RAND for their assistance with this report.

Contents

Figure and Tables

Figure

Tables

CHAPTER ONE

Background

Traumatic brain injuries (TBIs) and psychological health problems such as posttraumatic stress disorder (PTSD), depression, and substance use are common among U.S. military veterans who served in the era after September 11, 2001. These conditions are sometimes referred to as *invisible wounds* because they carry no physical marks but cause immense suffering for veterans and their families. Invisible wounds can interfere with veterans' employment, community engagement, relationships, and overall well-being (Tanielian and Jaycox, 2008; Trivedi et al., 2015). Although there are effective treatments for these conditions, many veterans with invisible wounds find it difficult to access high-quality care (Tanielian and Jaycox, 2008). In part, this is because it has been difficult for veterans, payers, and referring agencies to identify places that provide such care, as there has not been a shared definition of what makes care high quality. Defining high-quality care, identifying standards to benchmark care against the definition, and making this information available are essential for improving access to high-quality, effective care.

To address the challenges that veterans face when seeking care for invisible wounds, the George W. Bush Institute, a nonpartisan public policy arm of the George W. Bush Presidential Center, established the Veteran Wellness Alliance in 2017. The Veteran Wellness Alliance is a coalition of veteran peer-network and clinical provider organizations that aims to facilitate veterans' access to high-quality care for invisible wounds.[1] In support of this mission, the Bush Institute asked the RAND Corporation to establish a

---

[1] Additional information about the Veteran Wellness Alliance is available at George W. Bush Institute, undated (see https://www.bushcenter.org/veteran-wellness/index.html), and in Farmer and Dong, 2020.

definition of high-quality care for PTSD, depression, substance use, and TBI and to recommend corresponding standards of care. The goal of this effort was to improve the ability to identify high-quality care and facilitate access to such care for veterans who need it.

In the first phase of this work, we focused specifically on care for veterans with PTSD and TBI (Farmer and Dong, 2020). We proposed the following definition of high-quality care for these conditions based on four pillars: *High-quality care is veteran-centered, accessible, evidence-based, and includes outcome monitoring* (Figure 1.1).

- *Veteran-centered care* addresses the unique needs, values, and preferences of veterans by providing culturally competent care; assessing veterans' experience of care, including shared decisionmaking; and

FIGURE 1.1
Proposed Definition of High-Quality Care for Invisible Wounds

Veteran-centered	Accessible	Evidence-based	Includes outcome monitoring
• Provide culturally competent care • Assess veterans' care experience • Involve veterans in shared decisionmaking • Involve family and caregivers in treatment	• Ensure that care is timely • Reduce barriers to care	• Perform a comprehensive assessment • Provide psychotherapy and pharmaco-therapy according to clinical practice guidelines • Provide interdisciplinary team-based treatment • Perform appropriate screenings • Offer care coordination and treatment planning	• Use validated instruments to regularly assess clinical outcomes • Regularly assess other effects of care on life and well-being

involving family and caregivers (Farmer and Dong, 2020; Hamm et al., 2008; Institute of Medicine, 2001).

- *Accessible care* is timely and includes efforts to reduce barriers to care, including geographic, financial, and cultural barriers (Penchansky and Thomas, 1981).
- *Evidence-based care* is care that adheres to clinical practice guidelines—e.g., for PTSD (U.S. Department of Veterans Affairs [VA], 2017) and TBI (VA, 2021c)—and is based on empirical research demonstrating that a treatment or intervention is effective.
- *Outcome monitoring* is the routine administration of validated measurement tools (e.g., symptom rating scales) to assess patients' clinical outcomes from care. Outcome monitoring is a component of measurement-based care, in which health care providers use outcome data to guide clinical decisionmaking and collaborative treatment planning with patients (Fortney et al., 2017).

Although the definition is useful for establishing the essential tenets of high-quality care, operationalizing the definition through a set of standards of care can allow veterans, policymakers, providers, and payers to identify clinical providers who serve veterans and are currently delivering high-quality care. Standards of care are more specific than a definition (Minkoff, 2001) and, for our purpose, are intended to set a benchmark for what should be considered high-quality care. Standards of care can also provide a target for quality improvement: Providers who are not currently delivering high-quality care can identify gaps in the care they provide by comparing their care with the standards and implement necessary practice changes. To this end, we developed a set of standards of care that mapped to each pillar of high-quality care.

Methods

Before identifying standards of care, we first expanded the existing definition of high-quality care, which was initially limited to PTSD and TBI, to include care for depression and substance use (McLellan, 2017).[2] We did this to ensure that the high-quality care definition was useful across a variety of conditions under the umbrella of invisible wounds. We did not make any changes to the definition regarding the pillars of veteran-centered care and accessible care, as these are agnostic to a particular type of invisible wound and apply across conditions. To expand the definition regarding evidence-based care and outcome monitoring, we reviewed the academic and clinical literature on the treatment of depression and substance use, including VA and U.S. Department of Defense (DoD) clinical practice guidelines for these conditions (VA, 2016; VA, 2021a). We also conducted semistructured interviews with six clinical partners of the Veteran Wellness Alliance—representatives from the Cohen Veterans Network, the Marcus Institute for Brain Health, the SHARE Military Initiative at Shepherd Center, and the Warrior Care Network and two experts from the Veterans Health Administration (VHA)—to understand their approach to treating these two conditions and monitoring outcomes in veteran populations. The results of this synthesis are included in Appendix A.

Next, we used a collaborative process to operationalize the definition of high-quality care for invisible wounds into standards of care. Because these standards of care did not yet exist, we started by conducting a literature review of existing quality measures for PTSD, TBI, depression, and substance use, such as those endorsed by the National Quality Forum (NQF). We searched for quality measures because they focus on a specific aspect of care and can be used to measure the performance of health care providers (Centers for Medicare & Medicaid Services [CMS], 2021b). They are more specific than standards of care because they include a numerator and denominator and have strict mechanisms for collecting and scoring data. They are widely used by payers to distinguish between high- and low-performing providers and are an important source of information about what should be considered best practices, or standards of care. We organized existing quality measures according to the pillars of our high-quality care definition. We translated quality measures into standards of care by retaining the measure concept (e.g., veterans report that their provider communi-

---

[2] We defined *substance use* as including the spectrum of unhealthy use, from substance misuse to a substance use disorder (McLellan, 2017).

cated well) and setting aside specific details about inclusion and exclusion criteria and other aspects of the measure specification. Where no measures existed (for example, there is no existing measure of whether providers have received training in military cultural competence), we proposed a standard of care based on our expertise and previous research.

For standards of care to be useful, they must be both feasible and important. We assessed the feasibility of collecting data to demonstrate adherence with care standards through our interviews with Veteran Wellness Alliance clinical partners. In our interviews, we asked whether these programs had access to different data sources (e.g., patient surveys, medical records, administrative data) and whether they tracked certain types of information (type of psychotherapy provided, whether clinical providers had received training, etc.). We used this information to develop a list of potential standards of care that would be feasible and aligned with the definition of high-quality care.

We shared the list of standards of care with the Veteran Wellness Alliance peer-network and clinical partners, who rated each standard on its importance to the definition of high-quality care. We used this information to develop the set of recommended standards of care presented in this report. We describe these steps in more detail below.

Identification of Robust Potential Standards of High-Quality Care

We conducted a targeted literature review to identify existing scientific literature and reports describing existing quality measures in the context of general outpatient care delivery and for each of the conditions of interest (depression, PTSD, substance use disorder, and TBI). Specifically, we reviewed Mattox et al., 2016; Hepner et al., 2015; NQF-endorsed measures (NQF, 2021); CMS quality measures (CMS, 2021a); and the National Committee for Quality Assurance (NCQA) Healthcare Effectiveness Data and Information Set (HEDIS) measures (NCQA, 2021b). We also reviewed quality and performance measures currently used by VHA (Hussey et al., 2015). We abstracted each existing quality measure, corresponding data source(s), and operational definition as available. The literature review resulted in 97 quality measures across the four pillars: (1) veteran-centered care (n = 21),

(2) accessible care (n = 12), (3) evidence-based care (n = 45), and (4) care that includes outcome monitoring (n = 19). We translated each of these quality measures into standards of care and proposed an additional six standards of care for aspects of high-quality care for which we had found no existing measures.

Assessment of Feasibility of Potential Standards

We conducted semistructured interviews with clinical and administrative leadership from six organizations that provide care to veterans. Interviews were 30 minutes in length and were recorded, with permission of the interviewee, to help with reconciling our notes. During each interview, we discussed barriers to delivery of high-quality care for veterans, the role of standards of care, and potential strategies for assessing whether standards of care were met. We conducted an open-ended follow-up survey assessing interviewees' perspectives on potential standards of high-quality care (e.g., staff training in military cultural competence), whether they tracked this type of information already, and how feasible it would be to collect data if they did not already.

We synthesized information from the interviews and the survey to develop a definition of feasibility. We compiled interview notes into one document and looked for common themes about feasibility. We summarized survey responses, which provided greater detail about the feasibility of collecting specific types of data, including more-routine data (such as whether a patient screening had been conducted) and less-straightforward data (such as whether family members were included in treatment decisions). Together, the interviews and surveys provided a robust picture of which types of data clinical partners could reasonably collect quickly and which would take greater effort. In general, feasible data collection methods included extraction from administrative data sources and incorporation of additional questions in existing patient experience and symptom surveys. Data collection methods that required verbal assessment with patients, clinicians, or administrators were considered to be less feasible. Manual review of the electronic health record was generally considered to have relatively low feasibility, though interviewees provided feedback that some abstraction of data from medical records was feasible because they could automate abstraction or that similar fields were already routinely abstracted. Furthermore, some standards that could be assessed via medical record review could also be assessed by other mechanisms; for example, the standard for outcome measurement, "Percentage of veterans with TBI who have assessment of symptoms with NSI [Neurobehavioral Symptom Inventory] or other validated instrument during regular measurement periods," could be assessed by individual medical record review or by a clinic-level measure for clinics that have standardized care to require use of the NSI with all patients. Ultimately, data types were considered *feasible* if they used data that (1) were likely already being collected by organizations or (2) could easily be collected with existing data collection methods. Data types were considered burdensome if their feasibility was rated "low" in organizational feedback from interviews and post-interview surveys.

We used this information to narrow the initial set of standards of care identified in the literature review phase, resulting in a set of 33 potential standards of high-quality care.

Assessment of Importance of Potential Standards of Care

During the fall 2021 meeting of the Veteran Wellness Alliance, we presented the 33 proposed standards of care. We facilitated a discussion with leaders and representatives of Veteran Wellness Alliance partner organizations about the standards of care and reasonable goals for evaluating whether these standards were met in organizational and clinical practice. Subsequently, we asked Alliance representatives to provide written feedback on the relative importance of each the standards of care. We also asked them to comment on reasonable goals (i.e., the percentage of veterans who receive care that meets the standard) for each of the 33 standards of care (Appendix B). We asked respondents to rate each standard according to whether it was an important element of high-quality care (each standard was rated 1–10, where 1 was "not important at all" and 10 was "extremely important"). We consolidated the feedback from 14 respondents into mean importance ratings and summarized their qualitative feedback for each of the standards. We considered mean importance ratings of 8.0 or greater to be "highly rated" for importance.

Key Stakeholder Interviews

Finally, we conducted semistructured interviews with six VHA and Community Care Network representatives, one congressional staff member who works on veterans' issues, and two leaders of a veteran-serving organization about *whether* and *how* standards of care could be leveraged going forward. We selected these individuals based on their expertise in the field of veteran health care, their knowledge of quality standards, and our ability to contact them directly based on RAND's and the Bush Institute's network. Interviews were 30 minutes in length and were recorded, with permission of the interviewee, to help with reconciling our notes. We summarized themes from these interviews, identifying key similarities and differences reported by interviewees.

CHAPTER TWO

Proposed Standards of High-Quality Care for Invisible Wounds

As described in the previous chapter, we sought to operationalize the definition of high-quality care for veterans with invisible wounds by specifying standards of care. Our approach included an assessment of the feasibility of collecting data to demonstrate adherence to standards of care and consideration of the relative importance of potential standards.

Feasibility

We applied the feasibility criteria described in the previous section to the initial list of 103 potential high-quality care measures and standards. We identified 33 potential standards of care that would be feasible to collect based on data availability and program burden (Table 2.1). These standards represented care across the four pillars of high-quality care: veteran-centered (seven potential standards), accessible (four potential standards), evidence-based (two cross-cutting standards, three potential standards for depression, three potential standards for PTSD, five potential standards for substance use disorder, and four potential standards for TBI), and outcome monitoring (five potential standards).

Importance

Standards of care were considered *important* if clinicians and administrators rated them as a very important element of high-quality care (importance rating of 8.0 or greater). In general, standards were considered of low

TABLE 2.1

Potential Standards of Care for Invisible Wounds, Rated for Feasibility and Importance

Standard of Care	Data Type	Source	Aggregate Feasibility Rating	Mean Importance Rating	Included in Recommended Standards
Veteran-centered care					
1. Program/clinic staff have completed training in military cultural competence	Administrative data	RAND	High	8.2	Yes
2. Program/clinic staff have completed training in providing care to diverse groups of veterans	Administrative data	RAND	High	7.2	No
3. Veterans report that program/ clinic providers communicated well	Patient survey	AHRQ, 2016	Medium	7.2	No
4. Veterans report that they were involved as much as they wanted in the treatment they received from program/clinic	Patient survey	AHRQ, 2016	Medium	6.0	No
5. Veterans report that program/ clinic providers discussed including family and friends in their treatment	Patient survey	AHRQ, 2016	Medium	7.5	No
6. Veterans report being told about treatment options	Patient survey	AHRQ, 2016	Medium	9.2	Yes

Table 2.1—Continued

Standard of Care	Data Type	Source	Aggregate Feasibility Rating	Mean Importance Rating	Included in Recommended Standards
7. Program/clinic has staff who are knowledgeable about VA health care, including eligibility and enrollment and how to refer to/communicate with VA providers	Program self-report	Tanielian et al., 2018	Low	7.5	No
Accessible care					
8. Drive time to care within 30 minutes or program provides transportation	Administrative data	VA/Hussey et al., 2015	Medium	5.2	No
9. Veterans can schedule a new patient appointment/existing patient appointment within 30 days	Administrative data	VA/Hussey et al., 2015	High	7.6	Yes, revised: Veterans who request a new outpatient appointment can be seen within 30 days
10. Care is available at no or minimal cost to veterans: Program accepts insurance, has resources to support veterans without insurance, or is free	Administrative data	RAND	High	8.5	Yes

Table 2.1—Continued

Standard of Care	Data Type	Source	Aggregate Feasibility Rating	Mean Importance Rating	Included in Recommended Standards
11. Veterans report getting treatment quickly	Patient survey	AHRQ, 2016	High	6.3	No
Evidence-based care					
12. Veterans are assessed for suicide risk at each visit	Medical record	VA, 2021a	Medium	9.1	Yes
13. Veterans are assessed for recent substance use at each visit	Medical record	Hepner et al., 2015	Medium	7.9	No
14. (Depression) Veterans with depression with a newly prescribed antidepressant have a trial of 12 weeks	Medical record	NQF, 2021	Medium	5.3	No
15. (Depression) Veterans with depression receive evidence-based psychotherapy for depression[a]	Medical record	Hepner et al., 2015	Medium	9.2	Yes, combined with #18: Veterans with depression/ PTSD receive evidence-based psychotherapy for depression/PTSD

Table 2.1—Continued

Standard of Care	Data Type	Source	Aggregate Feasibility Rating	Mean Importance Rating	Included in Recommended Standards
16. (Depression) Veterans with depression receive at least four psychotherapy visits within the first 8 weeks of treatment	Administrative data	Hepner et al., 2015	High	7.3	No
17. (PTSD) Veterans with PTSD with a newly prescribed SSRI/SNRI have an adequate trial (≥60 days)	Medical record	Hepner et al., 2015	Medium	5.9	No
18. (PTSD) Veterans with PTSD receive evidence-based psychotherapy for PTSD[b]	Medical record	Hepner et al., 2015	Medium	9.2	Yes, combined with #15: Veterans with depression/PTSD receive evidence-based psychotherapy for depression/PTSD
19. (PTSD) Veterans with PTSD receive at least 4 psychotherapy visits within the first 8 weeks of treatment	Administrative data	Hepner et al., 2015	High	7.9	No

Table 2.1—Continued

Standard of Care	Data Type	Source	Aggregate Feasibility Rating	Mean Importance Rating	Included in Recommended Standards
20. (Substance use disorder) Veterans with substance use disorder are offered psychosocial intervention[c]	Medical record	Mattox et al., 2016	Medium	9.1	Yes
21. (Substance use disorder) Veterans with substance use disorder are offered pharmacotherapy	Medical record	Mattox et al., 2016	Medium	7.8	No
22. (Substance use disorder) Veterans with co-occurring mental health and substance use disorder receive integrated care for both conditions	Medical record	Mattox et al., 2016	High	8.8	Yes, combined with #27: Veterans with co-occurring conditions (mental health, substance use disorder, and/ or TBI) receive integrated care
23. (Substance use disorder) Veterans with substance use disorder initiate treatment within 14 days of diagnosis	Administrative data	NCQA, 2021b	High	6.6	No

Table 2.1—Continued

Standard of Care	Data Type	Source	Aggregate Feasibility Rating	Mean Importance Rating	Included in Recommended Standards
24. (Substance use disorder) Veterans who initiated treatment have two or more additional visits within 34 days of the initiation visit	Administrative data	NCQA, 2021b	High	6.7	No
25. (TBI) Program has a documented protocol including specific guidelines (e.g., Brain Trauma Foundation guidelines or institutional guidelines) for veterans with TBI	Program self-report	Carney et al., 2017	High	9.1	No
26. (TBI) Veterans with neurobehavioral deficits due to TBI receive appropriate treatment accommodations	Medical record	Substance Abuse and Mental Health Services Administration, 2021	Medium	9.2	No

Table 2.1—Continued

Standard of Care	Data Type	Source	Aggregate Feasibility Rating	Mean Importance Rating	Included in Recommended Standards
27. (TBI) Veterans with co-occurring mental health and TBI receive integrated care for both conditions	Medical record	VA, 2021c; Substance Abuse and Mental Health Services Administration, 2021	Medium	9.2	Yes, combined with #22: Veterans with co-occurring conditions (mental health, substance use disorder, and/or TBI) receive integrated care
28. (TBI) Program offers or facilitates multidisciplinary rehabilitation for veterans with TBI	Program self-report	VA, 2021c	Medium	8.4	Yes, revised: Program offers or facilitates coordinated, interdisciplinary rehabilitation for veterans with TBI
Outcome monitoring					
29. Program uses a validated instrument to regularly assess aspects of well-being (functioning, relationship quality, life satisfaction, etc.) at regular intervals (e.g., every 4 months)	Medical record	RAND	High	9.1	No

Table 2.1—Continued

Standard of Care	Data Type	Source	Aggregate Feasibility Rating	Mean Importance Rating	Included in Recommended Standards
30. (Depression) Percentage of veterans with depression with assessment of symptoms with PHQ-9 or other validated instrument during regular measurement periods (e.g., every 4 months)	Medical record	NQF, 2021	Medium	9.2	Yes, combined #30–33 into one measure: Program uses validated instruments to assess clinical symptoms during regular measurement periods (e.g., every 4 months)
31. (PTSD) Percentage of veterans with PTSD with assessment of symptoms with PCL-5 or other validated instrument during regular measurement periods (e.g., every 4 months)	Medical record	Hepner et al., 2015	Medium	9.3	

Table 2.1—Continued

Standard of Care	Data Type	Source	Aggregate Feasibility Rating	Mean Importance Rating	Included in Recommended Standards
32. (Substance use disorder) Percentage of veterans with substance use disorder with assessment of symptoms with BAM or other validated instrument during regular measurement periods (e.g., every 4 months)	Medical record	Mattox et al., 2016	Medium	9.3	Yes, combined #30–33 into one measure: Program uses validated instruments to assess clinical symptoms during regular measurement periods (e.g., every 4 months)
33. (TBI) Percentage of veterans with TBI who have assessment of symptoms with NSI, FIM, or other validated instrument during regular measurement periods (e.g., every 4 months)	Medical record	VA, 2021c	Medium	8.1	

NOTES: AHRQ = Agency for Healthcare Research and Quality; BAM = Brief Addiction Monitor; FIM = Functional Independence Measure; PCL-5 = PTSD Checklist for DSM–5; PHQ-9 = Patient Health Questionnaire-9; SNRI = serotonin and norepinephrine reuptake inhibitor; SSRI = selective serotonin reuptake inhibitor.

[a] Evidence-based psychotherapies for depression include acceptance and commitment therapy, behavioral therapy/behavioral activation, cognitive behavioral therapy (CBT), interpersonal therapy, mindfulness-based cognitive therapy, and problem-solving therapy.

[b] Evidence-based trauma-focused psychotherapies for PTSD include prolonged exposure, cognitive processing therapy, eye movement desensitization and reprocessing, CBT for PTSD, brief eclectic psychotherapy, narrative exposure therapy, and written exposure therapy.

[c] Psychosocial interventions for substance use disorder include behavioral couples therapy, CBT, the community reinforcement approach, motivational enhancement therapy, and 12-step facilitation.

importance if they were ambiguous or applied to only a subpopulation. Fourteen Veteran Wellness Alliance partners provided feedback on the importance of the standards. We report on the items that were assessed as very important in more detail below; these items were edited and consolidated into the final set of recommended standards.

Veteran-Centered Care

Of the seven potential standards of care associated with delivery of veteran-centered care, two were rated highly for importance:

- *Veterans report being told about treatment options* (importance rating: 9.2) received positive comments about its applicability in measuring guideline-concordant care, with acknowledgment that treatment options vary in appropriateness across patients and conditions. Comments also noted that the standard must allow for flexibility, with the understanding that such patient-reported items can be interpreted differently by patients, so they must be reasonably specific.
- *Program/clinic staff have completed training in military cultural competence* (importance rating: 8.2) received qualitative feedback that many clinical settings that serve veterans require military cultural competency training for staff, though a lack of systemic training in a clinic should not preclude patients from receiving care. One Veteran Wellness Alliance member stated, "While training per se is not a guarantee of a good outcome, a basic understanding of the military is necessary to establish rapport with a veteran or service member and to properly screen for appropriate exposures, experiences, and conditions."

Accessible Care

Four standards of care were associated with accessible care, and one was rated highly for importance. Another standard, rated lower, received qualitative feedback suggesting that it was highly important but should be revised:

- *Care is available at no or minimal cost to veterans* (importance rating: 8.5) had the caveat that out-of-pocket costs can be difficult to measure.

One Alliance member noted, "Cost can be a precluding factor, and so issues that participants have in covering the cost should be mitigated."

- *Veterans can schedule a new patient appointment/existing patient appointment within 30 days* (importance rating: 7.6) received feedback that wait time is an essential standard, though the goal should vary based on chronicity/usual care (e.g., within 14 or 30 days of referral) versus urgent conditions (e.g., within 12 hours). An Alliance partner stated, "Proposed goal of 'within 30 days' is reasonable for routine/new patient appointments; however, this should be less for more-urgent visits (mental health counseling, sickness)." Consistent with this feedback, some Alliance partners indicated that a standard goal shorter than 30 days was more appropriate (e.g., 14 days). Furthermore, appropriate wait times for intensive outpatient programs will necessarily be different from those for traditional outpatient treatment. Although some gave *average waiting time for a new patient appointment/existing patient appointment* a low score based on the proposed goal, the qualitative feedback strongly indicated that such a standard should be included with a revised goal.

Evidence-Based Care

Sixteen standards were associated with evidence-based care and rated high in importance, including one standard of general delivery of evidence-based care and 15 that were specific to one of the four conditions:

- *Veterans are assessed for suicide risk at each visit* (importance rating: 9.1) was highly endorsed, with qualitative emphasis on the importance of training and operationalization of this standard in clinical practice for clinics that care for veterans. One Alliance partner emphasized, "This is something we've learned the hard way. We should not forget those lessons when sending care out to the community. Training in how to assess should be part of the basic competency requirements."

For condition-specific evidence-based care, one pair of parallel standards was rated highly in importance for depression and PTSD:

- *Veterans with [depression/PTSD] receive evidence-based psychotherapy for [depression/PTSD]* (importance rating of 9.2 for both) received feedback that the standard should include caveats for psychotherapy being offered and declined by veterans and should exclude veterans for whom psychotherapy might not otherwise be appropriate. An Alliance partner stated of depression treatment, "We need to create incentives that encourage non-drug modalities which are appropriate even if drug treatment is also selected." We combined these depression and PTSD items for the final standard. This standard was additionally revised with consideration for pharmacotherapy, described in more detail in the next item.
- Of particular note, *Veterans with depression with a newly prescribed antidepressant have a trial of 12 weeks* (importance rating: 5.2) and *Percentage of veterans with PTSD with a newly prescribed SSRI/SNRI with an adequate trial (≥60 days)* (importance rating: 5.9) received low ratings and nuanced qualitative feedback. Qualitative feedback included concern for the specific guidance, emphasis on the importance of monitoring for adverse side effects, disagreements about how long medication trials should be, and concerns about the relationship between medication and psychotherapy, as summarized by this feedback: "If you choose to use an antidepressant, at least give it an adequate trial at an adequate dose with appropriate monitoring. However, I do have worries that this metric will encourage the use of drug as opposed to evidence-based psychotherapy." Based on such qualitative feedback, we instead incorporated the provision of evidence-based pharmacotherapy into a general treatment standard for depression and PTSD consistent with treatment guidelines: *Percentage of veterans with depression/PTSD who receive evidence-based psychotherapy and pharmacotherapy for depression/PTSD.*

Two standards of evidence-based care for substance use were highly rated:

- *Veterans are offered a psychosocial intervention for substance use disorder* (importance rating: 9.2) was highly rated, with emphasis that the standard should measure whether this service was offered rather than whether it was utilized, based on patient preferences for treatment.

- *Veterans with co-occurring mental health and substance use disorder receive integrated care for both conditions* (importance rating: 8.8) was also highly rated, with qualitative feedback that "integrated care" must be defined for effective interpretation of the standard. One Alliance partner emphasized, "It is critical that veterans with co-occurring mental health and substance use disorder receive integrated care for both conditions to ensure the veteran is receiving the most informed and comprehensive treatment to meet their unique needs."

Four standards of evidence-based care for TBI were rated high for importance:

- *Program has a documented protocol including specific guidelines for veterans with TBI* (importance rating: 9.1) received comments that clinical guidelines for TBI care in veterans remain less clear than those in other disease groups, and more research is necessary for care for veterans living with TBI. This feedback emphasized that the lack of clarity in protocols will make it too difficult to develop operational definitions for the standard. Based on this added feasibility feedback, we excluded the standard from the final set until stronger evidence is developed for TBI treatment guidelines.
- *Veterans with neurobehavioral deficits due to TBI receive appropriate treatment accommodations* (importance rating: 9.2) had feedback that "accommodations" should be defined. As in the previous item, feedback emphasized the difficulty in defining what accommodations should be made based on existing evidence and guidelines. Likewise, "appropriate" is difficult to operationalize in clinical guidance. Therefore, we also excluded this standard from the final set until guidelines define appropriate accommodations for TBI treatment.
- *Veterans with co-occurring mental health and TBI receive integrated care for both conditions* (importance rating: 9.2) similarly had feedback that "integrated" should be defined. An Alliance member commented, "All veterans with co-occurring mental health and TBI should receive integrated care for both conditions to ensure the veteran is receiving

the most informed and comprehensive care." Based on similar feedback and content, this item was consolidated with a parallel item (*Veterans with co-occurring mental health and substance use disorder receive integrated care for both conditions*) to become *Veterans with co-occurring conditions (e.g., mental health and substance use, mental health and TBI) receive integrated care.*

- *Program offers or facilitates multidisciplinary rehabilitation for veterans with TBI* (importance rating: 8.4) included qualitative feedback that "multidisciplinary rehabilitation" should be defined. Participants also acknowledged that not all clinical settings will have resources for multidisciplinary care. As one Alliance partner stated, "Programs should offer or facilitate multidisciplinary rehabilitation for veterans with TBI but if unable to, a referral should be made to an appropriate program or facility that is easily accessible." One Alliance partner commented that "programs should be interdisciplinary rather than multidisciplinary" and cautioned that "due to the complexity of the structural elements needed to ensure a basic level of quality, something like an accreditation pathway may be the best approach. You cannot rely simply on a check-box approach but have to assess whether the treatment plans are truly interdisciplinary." Based on feedback, we changed the wording of this standard from "multidisciplinary" to "interdisciplinary" and clarified that the program can facilitate interdisciplinary care if it does not have the resources to offer such care in its own clinical setting.

Outcome Monitoring

Five standards were associated with outcome monitoring, four of which were highly rated quantitatively for their importance and one of which was highly rated based on qualitative feedback:

- The general standard *Program uses validated instruments to regularly assess aspects of well-being (functioning, relationship quality, life satisfaction, etc.) at regular intervals (e.g., every four months)* (importance rating: 9.1) also received high endorsement in qualitative feedback, with emphasis that patient-reported well-being should be a primary goal of care. To that end, one Alliance partner said, "Should also include patient-reported outcomes, not just clinician administered scales." Another emphasized the importance of validated standards: "All programs must use validated instruments in assessments of well-being to ensure that what the clinician is intending to measure is actually being measured by the instrument." However, there are no existing instruments of well-being or functioning that are feasible to use, valid and reliable, and are sensitive to change (Hepner et al., 2021). Therefore, we did not include this standard in our recommended set of standards of care.

- The four parallel condition-specific standards of outcome monitoring were *Veterans with [condition] with assessment of symptoms with a validated instrument during regular measurement periods (e.g., every 4 months)* (importance ratings: 9.2 for depression, 9.3 for PTSD, 9.3 for substance use, and 8.1 for TBI) with specified examples of validated instruments in each group; qualitative feedback included that, while regular assessment is important, assessment could occur less frequently than the standard suggests because of patient factors. Further feedback included that some instruments are more well supported by experts than others, so validated instruments should be chosen thoughtfully. These four individual standards for depression, PTSD, substance use disorder, and TBI were combined for the final standard: *Program uses validated instruments to assess clinical symptoms during regular measurement periods (e.g., every 4 months)*. This standard provides a starting point by measuring whether a program is using a validated instrument; the next step for such outcome monitoring will include selection of specific instruments and measuring how frequently veterans are being assessed, whether programs are monitoring scores over time, and whether providers are using these data as part of shared decisionmaking and to inform treatment decisions.

Goal-Setting

Across the potential standards of care, Veteran Wellness Alliance partners who provided feedback emphasized that a goal of 100 percent for each standard of care (e.g., 100 percent of veterans reported being told about treatment options) was often unrealistic and that 80 percent or lower might be a more reasonable goal for many standards. Alliance partners cited several reasons for a reasonably lower goal, including a lack of necessity for high-quality care delivery for some standards (e.g., not all clinic staff need to receive military cultural competency training), a lack of clinical appropriateness in some cases (e.g., pharmacotherapy in conjunction with psychotherapy in treating invisible wounds is not always appropriate), veteran preferences for care (e.g., being offered but not choosing psychotherapy), and typical response rates for patient experience surveys. There is notable uncertainty about setting goals or thresholds for standards, and although we propose goals in Table 2.2, there is likely to be disagreement, warranting further discussion and research.

Recommended Standards of High-Quality Care

We selected a final set of ten standards of care, which were derived from the 33 potential standards of high-quality care. We aimed to select a parsimonious set of standards that addressed each of the pillars of high-quality care and all four conditions. We incorporated feedback from clinical providers, policymakers, and the diverse membership of the Veteran Wellness Alliance. Based on this feedback, we consolidated and edited standards for clarity, parsimony, and specificity and organized the ten recommended standards of care by the corresponding pillar of high-quality care (Table 2.2). The recommended standards are generally applicable across conditions, although specific standards of evidence-based care are included for depression, PTSD, substance use disorder, and TBI.

TABLE 2.2

Recommended Standards of High-Quality Care for Invisible Wounds

Standard Description	Proposed Performance Goal
Veteran-centered care	
Veterans report being told about treatment options	100 percent
Program/clinic staff who interact with veterans have completed training in military cultural competence	80 percent
Accessible care	
Care is available at no or minimal cost to veterans: Program accepts insurance, has resources to support veterans without insurance, or is free	Yes
Veterans who request a new outpatient appointment are seen within 30 days	80 percent
Evidence-based care	
Veterans are assessed for suicide risk at each visit	100 percent
Veterans with depression/PTSD receive evidence-based psychotherapy and/or pharmacotherapy for depression/PTSD[a,b]	80 percent
Veterans with substance use disorder are offered a psychosocial intervention[c]	80 percent
Veterans with co-occurring conditions (e.g., mental health and substance use, mental health and TBI) receive integrated care	80 percent
Program offers or facilitates coordinated, interdisciplinary rehabilitation for veterans with TBI	Yes
Outcome monitoring	
Program uses validated instruments to assess clinical symptoms during regular measurement periods (e.g., every 4 months)[d]	Yes

[a] Evidence-based psychotherapies for depression include acceptance and commitment therapy, behavioral therapy/behavioral activation, CBT, interpersonal therapy, mindfulness-based cognitive therapy, and problem-solving therapy.

[b] Evidence-based trauma-focused psychotherapies for PTSD include prolonged exposure, cognitive processing therapy, eye movement desensitization and reprocessing, CBT for PTSD, brief eclectic psychotherapy, narrative exposure therapy, and written exposure therapy.

[c] Psychosocial interventions for substance use disorder include behavioral couples therapy, CBT, the community reinforcement approach, motivational enhancement therapy, and 12-step facilitation. Psychosocial interventions are recommended for alcohol, cannabis, and stimulant use disorders. The evidence is unclear on the benefit of psychosocial interventions for opioid use disorder.

[d] Validated instruments include the PHQ-9 for depression (Kroenke, Spitzer, and Williams, 2001), the PCL-5 for PTSD (Weathers et al., 2013), the NSI (King et al., 2012) or FIM (Dodds et al., 1993) for TBI, and the BAM for substance use (Cacciola et al., 2013).

CHAPTER THREE

Implementing Standards of High-Quality Care: Insights from Policymakers

Current Efforts to Apply Quality Standards

Clinicians and administrators at Veteran Wellness Alliance clinical partner organizations outlined current efforts to apply quality care standards
to improve veteran outcomes. These interviewees discussed their existing
data collection efforts and the ways they use data to ensure high-quality
care delivery but noted that they currently do not report quality standards
for the care they provide to veterans. The exception to this is VHA, which
has a long-standing and robust approach to quality measurement, track-
ing and monitoring more than 500 quality and performance measures
across all types of clinical care, including 240 measures for mental health
care (Hussey et al., 2015). Clinical programs reported that they monitored
quality though regular meetings between care providers to discuss difficult
cases, review of cases by peers at regular intervals to check that protocols
and best practices were followed, and internal reporting on outcomes from
care. Many programs administer patient experience surveys to capture data
beyond medical outcomes.

Representatives from the VA Office of Community Care and VA Community Care Network contractors also discussed efforts to measure high-
quality care delivered by providers who contract with VA to provide care for
veterans. Under the VA MISSION Act of 2018, VA is required to establish
quality standards to be applied to both care delivered in VA facilities and
care provided outside VA by VA-contracted providers through the VA Com-

munity Care Network. While VHA has a robust quality measurement and reporting infrastructure for care delivered in VA facilities (Hussey et al., 2015), assessing the quality of VA Community Care Networks providers is in its infancy, and VA currently has no quality standards specific to veterans with behavioral health conditions or TBI (VA, 2021b).

VA Community Care Network contractors have begun to identify "high-performing providers" based on an algorithm that draws on a range of performance measures similar to some we discuss in this report. Community Care Network contractors identify and flag high-performing providers in their network, and VHA schedulers can use this information when scheduling appointments for veterans. VA is planning to include a high-performing provider designation on its external provider search website to enable veterans to identify high-performing Community Care Network providers. However, this system is not yet working as intended: When this report was finalized (late 2021), the high-performing provider algorithm had been applied to fewer than a quarter of all Community Care Network providers, and VHA schedulers were largely unaware of the existence of the high-performing provider flag.[1] Most importantly for identifying high-quality care for invisible wounds, behavioral health providers are not currently eligible for the "high-performing provider" designation in three of the five VA Community Care Network regions. In the two regions where behavioral health providers are eligible, the algorithm is based on Blue Health Intelligence Primary and Specialty Care measures, which are proprietary (we were unable to obtain information about what these include). Aside from the efforts to identify high-performing providers, representatives reported undergoing internal assessments using a range of measures, such as network adequacy (or the breadth of available services within network), drive time, and appointment availability.

---

[1] Personal communication with VA Office of Community Care personnel, 2021.

Barriers to Implementing and Reporting High-Quality Care Standards

Despite commitment from providers and payers to capture standards of high-quality care, barriers remain to implementing and reporting relevant standards. We summarize the most widely reported barriers here.

Data Quality and Availability

A commonly noted challenge to using high-quality care standards for behavioral health conditions and TBI was a lack of data to populate these standards. Some interviewees reported that the measures they use to track high quality are difficult to interpret. For example, one clinician reported that they tracked the number of veterans receiving a specific type of psychotherapy. However, the interviewee noted, this measure does not include how *much* therapy they are receiving. Without information on the volume of therapy, it was difficult to assess whether veterans were receiving high-quality care.

VA Office of Community Care representatives noted structural barriers to implementing our recommended standards of high-quality care for Community Care Network providers. First, the documentation that VA currently receives from network providers about the care that they provide to veterans is inadequate for assessing quality. Frequently, VA receives documentation that a veteran was seen by a network provider but no information about the treatment plan or what the care entailed—for example, whether an evidence-based psychotherapy was provided. Second, VA's contract with Community Care Network contractors does not require reporting on quality of care at the level of detail needed to populate our recommended standards. For example, network contractors are not required to report whether providers screen veterans for suicide risk, whether providers are trained in or provide evidence-based psychotherapy, or whether providers are trained in military cultural competence. However, Community Care Network contractor representatives noted that they collect information about provider certifications and credentials (which could include training in evidence-based psychotherapies), suggesting that this type of information could be reported if required by contract.

Tension Between Quality and Access

Programs and organizations that provide care to veterans must balance access to timely care with ensuring that the care provided is high quality. A key issue raised in our interviews was a lack of qualified providers capable of providing high-quality care to veterans with invisible wounds (i.e., depression, PTSD, substance use disorder, and TBI). For example, many providers in community care settings do not have training in evidence-based practices, particularly for mental health care. As VA Community Care Network contracts were developed, VA had extensive conversations about feasible expectations for community care providers and what trainings they could require. They were aware of the need to balance reasonable expectations so that community providers would participate with requirements for minimum standards to avoid low-quality care.[2] Even after considering such trade-offs, many requirements, such as requiring training in military cultural competence, were excluded from the contracts.

VA Community Care Network contractor representatives noted that, even without these requirements, it was difficult to recruit high-quality care providers within the network because providers view contracting with VA as more burdensome than with other payors (for example, there are documentation requirements to share medical records with VA). This is particularly true among providers for whom veterans make up only a small number of their patient population. One representative suggested that if contractors had more responsibility for case management (currently the referring VA provider has this responsibility), they would collect more information about the quality of care being provided—for example, by monitoring the effectiveness of psychotherapy and medication treatment. The representative noted that their organization collects some of this information for internal purposes already, even though it is not mandated by VA.

---

[2] Personal communication with VA Office of Community Care personnel, 2021.

Potential Solutions to Implementing High-Quality Care Standards

Increasing reimbursement for providers who successfully report (and eventually meet) a set of standards related to high-quality care for veterans, as outlined in this report, could increase the number of providers willing to adhere to such standards. Indeed, one policymaker suggested that our recommended standards could be used to align payer reimbursement with the delivery of high-quality care. One step short of that, payers could require that providers report on high-quality care standards and tie reimbursement to reporting.

Many organizations and payers already require some quality reporting; for example, CMS requires quality reporting through its Quality Payment Program. Because of these existing efforts, providers can use existing data and build on existing data collection mechanisms for many of the standards recommended in this report. Indeed, participants and policymakers indicated that administrative data and current patient-reported experience surveys could already provide data for many of our proposed standards.

CHAPTER FOUR

Recommendations

Currently, groups such as the Veteran Wellness Alliance, veterans, and payers face hurdles to identifying providers that provide high-quality care for veterans with depression, PTSD, substance use disorders, or TBI. There has been no agreed-upon standard by which to assess whether a provider or clinical program is high quality. Our goal was to create such a standard, or benchmark, to differentiate high- and low-quality care for these conditions.

The definition of high-quality care that we proposed in our first report (Farmer and Dong, 2020) and the recommended set of ten standards of high-quality care for invisible wounds outlined in this report could be used in multiple ways to improve the availability of high-quality care for veterans. To do this, first, the definition and standards should be shared with providers who treat veterans to set expectations for high-quality care. Second, providers who are not currently providing this level of care—for example, staff who have not been trained in military cultural competence or therapists who are not using evidence-based forms of psychotherapy—will need to start doing so, and they could need resources, incentives, or training. Third, providers will need to collect data to be able to report on specific metrics related to these standards and demonstrate that they are providing high-quality care.

Disseminate the Definition and Standards of High-Quality Care

The standards of care that we developed in this report can have impact both by identifying high-quality care providers and by encouraging other providers to improve care accordingly. The Veteran Wellness Alliance can encourage uptake within the Alliance and with other key stakeholder groups who serve veterans, including other provider coalitions, veteran service organizations, professional organizations, provider training programs, payers, VA, and Congress. Understanding standards (and applying quality measures when available) is the first step to robust outcome assessment and quality improvement.

Veteran service organizations can help to inform veterans and their families about what high-quality care is, how to ask for it, and how to find it. Professional organizations and provider training programs can tailor their certification requirements and curriculum to ensure that providers who serve veterans have the necessary training and resources to provide high-quality care for invisible wounds. Payers can use this to benchmark care and identify high-performing providers.

VA and Congress can use the recommended standards of high-quality care to inform the quality standards required by the VA MISSION Act for care delivered by VHA and the Community Care Network. Currently, VA's quality standards do not include measures for behavioral health care or TBI. In addition, VA Community Care Network contractors can use these standards to identify high-performing providers for behavioral health and TBI, enhancing the current approach that largely excludes providers who care for veterans with these conditions. With contractual changes, VA could require contractors to use these standards to inform identification of high-quality care providers for veterans in the Community Care Network. Given that 47 percent of all VA mental health care consultations are provided in the community,[1] ensuring that veterans are receiving high-quality care is a priority.

Broad dissemination of the definition and standards can improve veterans' outcomes by distinguishing high-quality care that meets these standards from other care that does not. This is especially true for evidence-based care. For example, new and innovative practices, such as those that incorporate building social capital or physical fitness or provide focus on personal growth, are popular and on the leading edge of interventions for PTSD, depression, substance use disorders, and TBI. Although these inter-

---

[1] Personal communication with VA Office of Community Care personnel, 2021.

ventions could prove to have clinical effectiveness, the research evidence at this point is limited. There are numerous, established approaches to treatment for invisible wounds that have been extensively researched and should always be used as the first line of treatment. As the field evolves in terms of evidence for additional treatments, a focus on evidence-based care as a key component of high-quality care will lead to better outcomes for veterans with invisible wounds. The same analogies can be applied to other aspects of the high-quality care definition.

Provide Resources and Incentives for Quality Improvement

Providers that serve veterans who do not currently meet the standards of high-quality care need to address gaps in quality, which will require a mix of feasible and compelling training, resources, and incentives.

Facilitate or Fund Training

Providers serving veterans with invisible wounds might need additional training to be able to provide care that meets the high-quality care standards. Trainings are available from multiple sources, including VA, nonprofit organizations serving the veteran community, and professional organizations, although most trainings have costs, which are sometimes significant.

VA offers trainings to VA Community Care Network providers, primarily via VHA TRAIN and seminars with the clinical community, though none are mandatory (VHA TRAIN, undated). Although a fair number of Community Care Network providers participate in the accessible trainings, participation is proportionally small (about 10 percent have completed training in military cultural competence) in comparison with the size of the entire Community Care Network.[2] This is evidence that simply offering training does not ensure engagement with or uptake of the training. VA provides additional trainings for VHA providers that are not available

---

[2] Personal communication with VA Office of Community Care personnel, 2021.

to community care providers, including health equity–based approaches to mental health needs.

Nonprofit organizations, such as PsychArmor, offer training in military culture for health care providers. The Center for Deployment Psychology at the Uniformed Services University offers training in evidence-based psychotherapies to clinicians serving military and veteran populations. Professional organizations, such as the National Association of Cognitive-Behavioral Therapists, offer training and certification in specific forms of evidence-based psychotherapies. Similar training and certifications exist for substance use disorder treatment approaches. Programs seeking to meet the standards of high-quality care can require that providers demonstrate competence in evidence-based forms of treatment by furnishing course transcripts, certificates, or other credentials. Although coursework does not necessarily indicate competence, such trainings provide a first, measurable step for competence. Financial support can buy time for clinicians to participate in training. Additionally, programs might need financial or administrative support for hosting trainings and facilitating providers' access to trainings.

Incentivize Quality Improvement

Currently, the standards of high-quality care that we have proposed are not required by payers or credentialing organizations. However, consortiums such as Veteran Wellness Alliance could use the ten standards we outline in this report to inform the selection of validated metrics that can eventually be used for reporting as a condition of membership. As an even more compelling incentive, payers could increase reimbursement rates or quality bonuses for high-quality care providers.

Start with a Minimum Set of Standards

While Veteran Wellness Alliance clinical partners would likely be able to use existing data to demonstrate that they meet each of the ten recommended standards, other providers may need to consider how to collect data to do this. For several standards, data collection could require adding additional questions to existing patient-experience surveys or adding fields to administrative databases. Although data for some standards might prove more challenging to collect than others, each was rated moderately or highly feasible because of the expected existing data collection infrastructure. That noted, it might be difficult for some providers to collect data for all ten standards of high-quality care without additional funding and resources.

To address this, we considered what standards should be required at a minimum to demonstrate that care was high quality. We identified three key standards that apply across the four conditions and represent each pillar of high-quality care:

- Demonstrating that veteran-facing clinical staff have received training in *military cultural competence* is critical. Just as providing culturally appropriate care is a tenet of all health care, specific military cultural competence training allows providers to consider the unique experiences, concerns, and values of veterans and better communicate with veterans about their goals and preferences for incorporation of those goals into care plans.
- Providers treating veterans with invisible wounds must demonstrate that the care they provide is *evidence-based*. To meet the standard, those who provide care for PTSD or depression must deliver an evidence-based psychotherapy or pharmacotherapy. Providers who treat veterans with substance misuse must offer a psychosocial intervention, and those who treat TBI must provide or facilitate interdisciplinary rehabilitation. Ideally, evidence-based care should also include regular monitoring of clinical symptoms with a validated instrument.
- Collecting data and reporting on *timeliness* to ensure that veterans seeking care can be seen by a provider within 30 days should be a requirement for programs providing high-quality care.

Although we believe that clinicians caring for veterans should aim to meet all ten of our high-quality care standards, we recommend these three as the minimum, essential set of standards that providers should meet to demonstrate that they provide high-quality care.

Considerations and Conclusion

We recognize that there are some complicating factors to implementing and demonstrating that the standards of high-quality care have been met. For instance, heterogeneity in veteran populations adds to the complexity of setting goals for some of the standards. In some cases, expectations for care and veterans' involvement with treatment decisionmaking could vary depending on treatment options and veteran preferences. For example, goals for the delivery of high-quality, evidence-based care might vary by the approach preferred by the veteran (e.g., pharmacotherapy versus psychotherapy). There is also a need for more evidence in some areas, such as TBI, where quality measures have not yet been standardized and the range of evidence-based treatment approaches is broad. Although we included four conditions in our current set of standards, more work is necessary to expand the definition and standards to other conditions that impact veterans.

Not all providers will be able to meet the standards of care set out in this report immediately. There must be some flexibility as care providers raise the quality of care and upskill to address gaps in their care. In setting goals, we recommend identifying what is achievable and nonnegotiable, such as the provision of evidence-based care. Other requirements will be initially aspirational, and, as such, organizations can select thresholds for improvement over time that make sense based on the starting point of the provider. We also recognize that there is a tension between requiring care to meet these standards and ensuring that veterans are able to access needed care. Adding administrative burden to providers could dissuade them from serving veterans, reducing the pool of high-quality care providers. In some geographic areas, there might be too few providers to ensure that all veterans who need care receive it from a provider that can demonstrate their ability to meet the high-quality care standards outlined here. In these cases, requiring providers to meet minimum standards could systematically reduce access in inequitable ways (e.g., disproportionately reducing access in rural and other underserved areas). Extending opportunities for telehealth and other technological solutions could help to bridge the gap to high-quality care across geography and veteran populations.

Limitations

The standards of care presented in this report should be interpreted with consideration of several limitations. First, our interviews included a relatively small number of people. Although we sought diverse perspectives among our participants, the views herein, including those from Veteran Wellness Alliance members, are not representative of all veteran care providers. Second, assessments of feasibility were drawn from a set of clinical providers that could have access to more resources and more-sophisticated data infrastructure than the average clinical provider. As noted above, less well-resourced providers might find that demonstrating that they meet the recommended standards of care requires additional resources to collect the needed data. Finally, the goals suggested for each standard of care are not based on data and analysis but rather are informed by expert opinion. Future work to refine these goals should examine variability in providers' progress toward these notional goals (e.g., determine what percentage of veterans are currently receiving care according to these standards) to identify achievable and meaningful actual goals.

Next Steps

To assess whether programs that provide care for veterans meet the recommended standards of care, the Veteran Wellness Alliance or other entities might wish to create a checklist to enable programs to self-report, using available data, their progress on each of the standards of care. This checklist could be piloted with a few programs to ensure that directions are clear on what kind of data or evidence should be provided along with the self-report (for example, programs might be asked to provide documentation on provider training in military cultural competence).

The development and dissemination of standards of high-quality care for invisible wounds is a crucial step toward improving access to high-quality care for veterans. Future steps could include the development and implementation of specific quality or performance measures, which would allow measurement by accrediting entities or payors of the quality of care provided for invisible wounds, comparison across providers, and a standardized approach to quality reporting. For some standards of care, there are existing quality measures that have been fully developed and tested for reliability and validity (e.g., measures that have been endorsed by NQF or are in use by federal health care quality reporting programs, such as HEDIS). For many other standards, however, investments in measure development would be required, as no fully developed measures currently exist. De novo measure development would require additional engagement of programs and providers that care for veterans and engagement with measure developers.

Conclusion

This report recommends ten standards of care to operationalize the definition of high-quality care for veterans with invisible wounds. Adoption of these standards of care would allow veterans, veteran-serving organizations, and payers to identify high-quality care providers and distinguish between good and poor care. The standards also provide a road map for providers that fall short of the benchmark and might need to invest in training and other resources to improve quality and demonstrate their ability to provide the best possible care for veterans living with invisible wounds.

Evidence-Based Care for Depression and Substance Use Disorders

To ensure that the high-quality care definition was useful across a variety of conditions under the umbrella of invisible wounds, we expanded the existing definition of high-quality care, which was initially limited to PTSD and TBI, to include care for depression and substance use disorders. Evidence-based care generally includes performance of a comprehensive assessment, provision of psychotherapy and pharmacotherapy according to clinical practice guidelines, provision of interdisciplinary team-based treatment, and offer of care coordination and treatment planning. However, aspects of evidence-based care are condition-specific. Our review of evidence-based care for PTSD and TBI was published in a previous report (Farmer and Dong, 2020). Here, we report results of our review of evidence-based care for depression and substance use disorders.

For this review, we conducted a targeted literature review strategy. We started with the most recent VA clinical practice guidelines for treatment. We then searched the literature for evaluations of the recommended pharmacotherapy, psychotherapy, and psychosocial interventions for depression and substance use disorders to develop a more detailed understanding of the efficacy of these interventions among veterans. We primarily relied on PubMed and Google Scholar for our literature search.

Depression

The VA/DoD clinical practice guideline for the management of major depressive disorder (MDD; depression) (VA, 2016) recommends offering either evidence-based psychotherapy or evidence-based pharmacotherapy as a first-line treatment for uncomplicated mild to moderate depression.[1] Evidence-based psychotherapeutic techniques include (1) acceptance and commitment therapy, (2) behavioral therapy/behavioral activation, (3) CBT, (4) interpersonal therapy, (5) mindfulness-based cognitive therapy, and (6) problem-solving therapy (Hundt et al., 2014).

Recommended pharmacotherapies include SSRIs (except fluvoxamine), SNRIs, mirtazapine, and bupropion (VA, 2016). Guidelines suggest that providers engage with patients and discuss safety and the side-effect profile, history of prior response to a particular medication, family history of response to a medication, concurrent medical illnesses, concurrently prescribed medications, the cost of the medication, and provider training and competence to determine which intervention best meets the patient's needs (Puetz, Youngstedt, and Herring, 2015).

While evidence-based approaches for treating depression are well established, the current research does not yet support the use of a particular evidence-based psychotherapy or pharmacotherapy over another. For patients who have had a partial response or no response to a single initial pharmacotherapy after a minimum of four to six weeks, the guideline recommends switching to another therapy (medication or psychotherapy) or augmenting the first pharmacotherapy treatment approach with a second medication or psychotherapy. For patients who select psychotherapy as a treatment option, the guideline suggests offering individual or group-based psychotherapy, depending on patient preferences. For patients with mild to moderate depression, the guideline recommends supplementing the initial treatment with computer-based CBT or, depending on patient preferences, offering this type of therapy as a first-line treatment. Likewise, telehealth (e.g., video or telephone visits) and collaborative care (e.g., access to special-

---

[1]   An update to the VA/DoD Clinical Practice Guideline for the Management of Major Depressive Disorder was in progress when this report was finalized in late 2021 but had not yet been published.

ists via their collaboration with primary care) offer opportunities to improve access to VA psychotherapy services, including in rural areas (Fortney et al., 2012; Fortney et al., 2007).

Although there is variability in types of psychotherapy that are delivered for depression, CBT is the most commonly used evidence-based psychotherapy for depression. Even when evidence-based psychotherapy is delivered, whether it is delivered with fidelity is rarely assessed, particularly for care delivered outside VA clinical jurisdiction (Schlosser et al., 2020). Within VA, use of evidence-based psychotherapy for the treatment of depression is improving given the internal emphasis on such services (Mott et al., 2014), although there are disparities in access to evidence-based psychotherapy for rural veterans (Cully et al., 2010).

Summary of Veteran Wellness Alliance Partner Interviews

As described earlier in this report, we conducted interviews with Veteran Wellness Alliance clinical partners to understand their approach to treating depression among veterans. Most interviewees reported that treatment starts with a biopsychosocial assessment to determine or confirm the veteran's depression diagnosis. One interviewee stressed the importance of this step because getting the right diagnosis is paramount and can be difficult as veterans can present with multiple invisible wounds. Following this assessment, most Alliance providers deliver CBT as the primary treatment approach for veterans with depression.

One clinical provider described using two therapy modalities, individual and group therapy. Individual therapy took place at least once a week, and group therapy occurred less frequently but included emotional regulation education. Some providers offered classes in addition to CBT to strengthen coping strategies, teach diaphragmatic breathing, and offer practical approaches to managing depression. Another provider noted that they augmented CBT with other approaches, such as art therapy.

Veteran Wellness Alliance clinical partners reported working with physicians to determine appropriate medication treatment. One interviewee noted that they rarely prescribe medications themselves but will connect a patient to a local psychiatrist who can support them if needed.

Substance Use Disorders

The VA/DoD clinical practice guideline for the management of substance use disorder (VA, 2021a) recommends a range of both pharmacotherapy and behavioral interventions. To address alcohol misuse, the guidelines recommend screening regularly using the three-item Alcohol Use Disorders Identification Test—Consumption or the Single-Item Alcohol Screening Questionnaire. The guidelines also suggest benzodiazepines with monitoring for moderate to severe alcohol withdrawal. To treat moderate to severe alcohol use disorder, the guidelines suggest pharmacotherapy with naltrexone or topiramate. For patients in early recovery or relapse of alcohol misuse, the guidelines recommend promoting involvement in a mutual help program, such as 12-step facilitation (VA, 2021a).

For alcohol misuse that does not meet diagnostic criteria for alcohol use disorder, the recommended first-line treatment is known as Screening, Brief Intervention, and Referral to Treatment (Babor et al., 2007). Brief interventions focus on discussions of alcohol-related risks and physician recommendations to abstain from alcohol (Moyer, 2013). This approach has been adopted in primary care and mental health clinics and is being increasingly adopted in military populations (Ahmadi and Green, 2011; Harris and Yu, 2019; Holt et al., 2017). If patients do not respond to brief behavior change intervention alone, they should be referred to specialty behavioral health clinics for more-intensive pharmacological or psychosocial treatment.

For opioid use disorder, the guideline recommends pharmacotherapy with buprenorphine or naloxone and methadone in inpatient or accredited treatment program settings (VA, 2021a). Patients with sedative hypnotic use disorder should gradually taper with benzodiazepines for withdrawal management. Patients with cocaine use disorder are recommended to use one of the following psychosocial interventions: CBT, recovery-focused behavioral therapy, or contingency management in combination with another behavioral intervention. As with alcohol misuse, the guidelines suggest that patients with drug use disorders in early recovery or following relapse become involved in group mutual health programs, such as peer linkage or 12-step facilitation. These treatment options have a strong evidence base in both the general population and veterans (Teeters et al., 2017).

For all substances, the guideline provides recommendations for addiction-focused medication management, including monitoring adherence, response to treatment, and adverse effects; educating patients about the health consequences of substance use and possible treatments; encouraging patients to abstain from illicit opioids and other addictive substances; encouraging referrals to community support for recovery and patients' subsequent attendance; and encouraging patients to make lifestyle changes that support recovery.

Primary care and psychotherapy settings can often provide education and supplementary support to veterans living with unhealthy substance use. However, many care settings are not equipped to treat substance use disorder and require collaboration with specialty facilities.

Unhealthy substance use often co-occurs with other behavioral and mental health conditions, and substances are indeed often used as self-management of other symptoms, including insomnia. Therefore, concurrent treatment for both substance use and mental health conditions is recommended, rather than requiring management of substance use prior to enrollment in other treatment programs. The shift to concurrent care of substance use disorder and other conditions facilitates more veteran-centered care, though additional research is necessary to determine best practices and models for such interconnected care (Smucker, Pedersen, and Tanielian, 2019).

The most recent VA/DoD guideline (VA, 2021a) also discusses the importance of telehealth. While evidence of the effectiveness of telehealth options for substance use disorders is still developing, there is evidence that using technology-based interventions such as automated text or voice messaging and smartphone apps in addition to usual care could support patients with alcohol use disorder (but it is unclear whether this is helpful for other substance use disorders) (VA, 2021a). Structured telephone-based care in addition to usual care for substance use disorders can also support patients (VA, 2021a). However, it is too soon to tell whether other computer-based health care services are helpful for patients with substance use disorders.

Summary of Interviews with Veteran Wellness Alliance Partners

Most Veteran Wellness Alliance clinical providers reported that they do not treat substance use disorders. Instead, most reported sending veterans to other providers for help with substance use prior to initiating treatment for mental health conditions. One interviewee reported that they would provide mental health care for veterans with co-occurring substance use disorder, though another indicated that they wanted veterans to maintain sobriety for six months prior to entering the facility. This provider noted that they were currently studying whether they could accept veterans with substance use problems into their treatment program, as they recognize that co-occurring substance use disorders are one of the main barriers to care for other invisible wounds, such as PTSD and TBI.

VHA representatives reported that VHA substance use treatment focuses on contingency management, CBT, and harm reduction. VHA providers use both pharmacotherapy (pharmacotherapy with buprenorphine or naloxone and methadone in inpatient or accredited treatment program settings) and psychotherapy and psychosocial treatment, depending on the substance type, severity, and other patient factors.

Standards of Care Assessed for Importance

Veteran Wellness Alliance partners were asked to provide feedback on 33 potential standards of care with the following instructions:

1. Please rate each standard on a scale of 1 (not important at all) to 10 (extremely important) and include notes on your thoughts and reactions about which of these items are important to measure.
2. Please provide notes on whether the proposed goal is reasonable or offer alternative suggestions.

Table B.1 provides the original phrasing of the standards as they were assessed by Veteran Wellness Alliance partners and proposed goals. Participants were given open-ended space to provide their importance rating on a scale of 1 to 10, describe their importance rating, and provide other comments or considerations.

TABLE B.1

Potential Standards of High-Quality Care Assessed for Importance by Veteran Wellness Alliance Partners

Standard of Care Statement	Proposed Goal
Quality pillar: Care is veteran-centered	
1. Percentage of program/clinic staff who completed training in military cultural competence	100%
2. Percentage of program/clinic staff who completed training in providing care to diverse groups of veterans	100%
3. Percentage of veterans who report that program/clinic providers communicated well	100%
4. Percentage of veterans who report that they were involved as much as they wanted in the treatment they received from program/clinic	100%
5. Percentage of veterans who report that program/clinic providers discussed including family and friends in their treatment	100%
6. Percentage of veterans who report being told about treatment options	100%
7. Program/clinic has staff who are knowledgeable about VA health care, including eligibility and enrollment and how to refer to/communicate with VA providers	Yes
Quality pillar: Care is accessible	
8. Average travel distance (driving time) for veterans	Within 30 minutes OR program provides transportation
9. Average waiting time for a new patient appointment/existing patient appointment	Within 30 days
10. Average out of pocket cost for treatment	Minimal financial burden: accept insurance; have resources to support veterans without insurance
11. Percentage of veterans who report getting treatment quickly	100%

Table B.1—Continued

Standard of Care Statement	Proposed Goal
Quality pillar: Care is evidence-based	
12. Percentage of veterans assessed for suicide risk at each visit	100%
13. Percentage of veterans assessed for recent substance use at each visit	100%
Evidence-based care for major depressive disorder (MDD)	
14. Percentage of veterans with MDD with a newly prescribed antidepressant with a trial of 12 weeks	100%
15. Percentage of veterans with MDD who receive evidence-based psychotherapy for depression	100%
16. Percentage of veterans with MDD who receive at least 4 psychotherapy visits within the first 8 weeks of treatment	100%
Evidence-based care for posttraumatic stress disorder (PTSD)	
17. Percentage of veterans with PTSD with a newly prescribed SSRI/SNRI with an adequate trial ($\geq$60 days)	100%
18. Percentage of veterans with PTSD who receive evidence-based psychotherapy for PTSD	100%
19. Percentage of veterans with PTSD who receive at least 4 psychotherapy visits within the first 8 weeks of treatment	100%
Evidence-based care for substance use disorder (SUD)	
20. Percentage of veterans who are offered psychosocial intervention for substance misuse (12-step programs, cognitive behavioral therapy, motivational enhancement therapy, brief alcohol interventions, aftercare components, contingency management, work therapy, other psychosocial interventions)	100%
21. Percentage of veterans who are offered pharmacotherapy for SUD (disulfiram, naltrexone, fluoxetine, paroxetine, desiramine, sertraline, lamotrigine, aripiprazole, lithium, topiramate, prazosin, other pharmacologic options)	100%
22. Percentage of veterans with co-occurring mental health and SUD who receive integrated care for both conditions	100%

Table B.1—Continued

Standard of Care Statement	Proposed Goal
23. Percent of veterans with SUD who initiated treatment within 14 days of diagnosis through an inpatient AOD admission, outpatient visit, intensive outpatient encounter or partial hospitalization, telehealth or medication-assisted treatment (MAT)	100%
24. Percentage of veterans who initiated treatment and had two or more additional SUD services or MAT within 34 days of the initiation visit	100%
Evidence-based care for traumatic brain injury (TBI)	
25. Program has a documented protocol including specific guidelines (e.g., Brain Trauma Foundation guidelines or institutional guidelines) for veterans with TBI (yes/no)	Yes
26. Percentage of veterans with neurobehavioral deficits due to TBI who receive appropriate treatment accommodations	100%
27. Percentage of veterans with co-occurring mental health and TBI who receive integrated care for both conditions	100%
28. Program offers or facilitates multidisciplinary rehabilitation for veterans with TBI (yes/no)	Yes
Quality pillar: Care includes outcome monitoring	
29. Program uses a validated instrument to regularly assess aspects of well-being (functioning, relationship quality, life satisfaction, etc.) at regular intervals (e.g., every 4 months) (e.g., LISAT 11, VR-12, SF-36)	Yes
30. Percentage of veterans with MDD with assessment of symptoms with PHQ-9 or other validated instrument during regular measurement periods (e.g., every 4 months)	100%
31. Percentage of veterans with PTSD with assessment of symptoms with PCL or other validated instrument during regular measurement periods (e.g., every 4 months)	100%
32. Percentage of veterans with SUD with assessment of symptoms with AUDIT, CAGE, or other validated instrument during regular measurement periods (e.g., every 4 months)	100%
33. Percentage of veterans with TBI who have assessment of symptoms with NSI or other validated instrument during regular measurement periods (e.g., every 4 months)	100%

NOTES: AOD = alcohol and other drug; AUDIT= Alcohol Use Disorders Identification Test; CAGE = CAGE Alcohol Questionnaire; LISAT 11 = Life Satisfaction Questionnaire 11; SF-36 = 36-Item Short-Form Health Survey; VR-12 = Veterans RAND 12-Item Health Survey.

Abbreviations

AHRQ	Agency for Healthcare Research and Quality
AOD	alcohol and other drug
AUDIT	Alcohol Use Disorders Identification Test
BAM	Brief Addiction Monitor
CAGE	CAGE Alcohol Questionnaire
CBT	cognitive behavioral therapy
CMS	Centers for Medicare & Medicaid Services
DoD	U.S. Department of Defense
FIM	Functional Independence Measure
HEDIS	Healthcare Effectiveness Data and Information Set
LISAT 11	Life Satisfaction Questionnaire 11
MDD	major depressive disorder
NCQA	National Committee for Quality Assurance
NQF	National Quality Forum
NSI	Neurobehavioral Symptom Inventory
PCL-5	PTSD Checklist for DSM–5
PHQ-9	Patient Health Questionnaire-9
PTSD	posttraumatic stress disorder
SF-36	36-Item Short-Form Health Survey
SNRI	serotonin and norepinephrine reuptake inhibitor
SSRI	selective serotonin reuptake inhibitor
TBI	traumatic brain injury
VA	U.S. Department of Veterans Affairs
VHA	Veterans Health Administration
VR-12	Veterans RAND 12-Item Health Survey

References

Agency for Healthcare Research and Quality, *CAHPS ECHO Survey Measures*, Rockville, Md., May 2016, last updated May 2018. As of December 3, 2021: https://www.ahrq.gov/cahps/surveys-guidance/echo/about/survey-measures.html

Ahmadi, Halima, and Scott L. Green, "Screening, Brief Intervention, and Referral to Treatment for Military Spouses Experiencing Alcohol and Substance Use Disorders: A Literature Review," *Journal of Clinical Psychology in Medical Settings*, Vol. 18, No. 2, 2011, pp. 129–136.

AHRQ—*See* Agency for Healthcare Research and Quality.

Babor, Thomas F., Bonnie G. McRee, Patricia A. Kassebaum, Paul L. Grimaldi, Kazi Ahmed, and Jeremy Bray, "Screening, Brief Intervention, and Referral to Treatment (SBIRT): Toward a Public Health Approach to the Management of Substance Abuse," *Journal of Substance Abuse Treatment*, Vol. 28, No. 3, 2007, pp. 7–30.

Cacciola, John S., Arthur I. Alterman, Dominick Dephilippis, Michelle L. Drapkin, Charles Valadez Jr, Natalie C. Fala, David Oslin, and James R. McKay, "Development and Initial Evaluation of the Brief Addiction Monitor (BAM)," *Journal of Substance Abuse Treatment*, Vol. 44, No. 3, March 2013, pp. 256–263.

Carney, Nancy, Annette M. Totten, Cindy O'Reilly, Jamie S. Ullman, Gregory W. Hawryluk, Michael J. Bell, Susan L. Bratton, Randall Chesnut, Odette A. Harris, Niranjan Kissoon, and Andres M. Rubiano, Lori Shutter, Robert C. Tasker, Monica S. Vavilala, Jack Wilberger, David W. Wright, and Jamshid Ghajar, "Guidelines for the Management of Severe Traumatic Brain Injury," *Neurosurgery*, Vol. 80, No. 1, January 1, 2017, pp. 6–15.

Centers for Medicare & Medicaid Services, "Measures Inventory Tool," homepage, June 30, 2021a. As of December 3, 2021: https://cmit.cms.gov/CMIT_public/ListMeasures

Centers for Medicare & Medicaid Services, "What Is a Quality Measure?" webpage, last updated December 1, 2021b. As of December 3, 2021: https://www.cms.gov/Medicare/Quality-Initiatives-Patient-Assessment-Instruments/MMS/NTM-What-is-a-Quality-Measure-SubPage

CMS—*See* Centers for Medicare & Medicaid Services.

Cully, Jeffrey A., John P. Jameson, L. L. Phillips, Mark E. Kunik, and John C. Fortney, "Use of Psychotherapy by Rural and Urban Veterans," *Journal of Rural Health*, Vol. 26, No. 3, Summer, 2010, pp. 225–233.

Dodds, T. Andrew, Diane P. Martin, Walter C. Stolov, and Richard A. Deyo, "A Validation of the Fuctional Independence Measurement and Its Performance Among Rehabilitation Inpatients," *Archives of Physical Medicine and Rehabilitation*, Vol. 74, No. 5, May 1993, pp. 531–536.

Farmer, Carrie M., and Lu Dong, *Defining High-Quality Care for Posttraumatic Stress Disorder and Mild Traumatic Brain Injury: Proposed Definition and Next Steps for the Veteran Wellness Alliance*, Santa Monica, Calif.: RAND Corporation, RR-A337-1, 2020. As of December 3, 2021: https://www.rand.org/pubs/research_reports/RRA337-1.html

Fortney, John, Mark Enderle, Skye McDougall, Jeff Clothier, Jay Otero, and Lisa Altman, "Implementation Outcomes of Evidence-Based Quality Improvement for Depression in VA Community Based Outpatient Clinics," *Implementation Science*, Vol. 7, April 11, 2012, p. 30.

Fortney, John C., Jeffrey M. Pyne, Mark J. Edlund, David K. Williams, Dean E. Robinson, Dinesh Mittal, and Kathy L. Henderson, "A Randomized Trial of Telemedicine-Based Collaborative Care for Depression," *Journal of General Internal Medicine*, Vol. 22, No. 8, 2007, pp. 1086–1093.

Fortney, John C., Jürgen Unützer, Glenda Wrenn, Jeffrey M. Pyne, Richard G. Smith, Michael Schoenbaum, Henry T. Harbin, "A Tipping Point for Measurement-Based Care," *Psychiatric Services*, Vol. 68, February 1, 2017, pp. 179–188.

George W. Bush Institute, "Veteran Wellness Alliance," webpage, undated. As of January 10, 2022: https://www.bushcenter.org/veteran-wellness/index.html

Hamm, William G., Virginia T. Betts, Dennis M. Duffy, Frank A. Fairbanks, Thomas L. Garthwaite, Donald F. Kettl, Bernard D. Rostker, and Daniel L. Skoler, *After Yellow Ribbons: Providing Veteran-Centered Services*, Washington, D.C.: National Academy of Public Administration, No. 2116, 2008.

Harris, Brett R., and Jiang Yu, "Service Access and Self-Reporting: Tailoring SBIRT to Active Duty Military in Civilian Health Care Settings," *Journal of Social Work Practice in the Addictions*, Vol. 19, No. 1–2, April 3, 2019, pp. 177–187.

Hepner, Kimberly A., Carol P. Roth, Coreen Farris, Elizabeth M. Sloss, Grant R. Martsolf, Harold Alan Pincus, Katherine E. Watkins, Caroline Batka, Daniel Mandel, Susan D. Hosek, and Carrie M. Farmer, *Measuring the Quality of Care for Psychological Health Conditions in the Military Health System: Candidate Quality Measures for Posttraumatic Stress Disorder and Major Depressive Disorder*, Santa Monica, Calif.: RAND Corporation, RR-464-OSD, 2015. As of December 3, 2021: https://www.rand.org/pubs/research_reports/RR464.html

Hepner, Kimberly A., Carol P. Roth, Heather Krull, Lea Xenakis, and Harold Alan Pincus, *Readiness of Soldiers and Adult Family Members Who Receive Behavioral Health Care: Identifying Promising Outcome Metrics*, Santa Monica, Calif.: RAND Corporation, RR-4268-A, 2021. As of November 16, 2021: https://www.rand.org/pubs/research_reports/RR4268.html

Holt, Megan, Mark Reed, Susan I. Woodruff, Gerard DeMers, Michael Matteucci, and Suzanne L. Hurtado, "Adaptation of Screening, Brief Intervention, Referral to Treatment to Active Duty Military Personnel in an Emergency Department: Findings from a Formative Research Study," *Military Medicine*, Vol. 182, No. 7, 2017, pp. e1801–e1807.

Hundt, Natalie E., Terri L. Barrera, Andrew Robinson, and Jeffrey A. Cully, "A Systematic Review of Cognitive Behavioral Therapy for Depression in Veterans," *Military Medicine*, Vol. 179, No. 9, 2014, pp. 942–949.

Hussey, Peter S., Jeanne S. Ringel, Sangeeta C. Ahluwalia, Rebecca Anhang Price, Christine Buttorff, Thomas W. Concannon, Susan L. Lovejoy, Grant R. Martsolf, Robert S. Rudin, Dana Schultz, Elizabeth M. Sloss, Katherine E. Watkins, Daniel A. Waxman, Melissa Bauman, Brian Briscombe, James R. Broyles, Rachel M. Burns, Emily K. Chen, Amy Soo Jin DeSantis, Liisa Ecola, Shira H. Fischer, Mark W. Friedberg, Courtney A. Gidengil, Paul B. Ginsburg, Timothy R. Gulden, Carlos Ignacio Gutierrez Gaviria, Samuel Hirshman, Christina Y. Huang, Ryan Kandrack, Amii M. Kress, Kristin J. Leuschner, Sarah MacCarthy, Ervant J. Maksabedian Hernandez, Sean Mann, Luke J. Matthews, Linnea Warren May, Nishtha Mishra, Lisa Kraus, Ashley N. Muchow, Jason Nelson, Diana Naranjo, Claire E. O'Hanlon, Francesca Pillemer, Zachary Predmore, Rachel Ross, Teague Ruder, Carolyn M. Rutter, Lori Uscher-Pines, Mary E. Vaiana, Joseph Vesely, Susan D. Hosek, and Carrie M. Farmer, *Resources and Capabilities of the Department of Veterans Affairs to Provide Timely and Accessible Care to Veterans*, Santa Monica, Calif.: RAND Corporation, RR-1165/2-VA, 2015. As of December 3, 2021: https://www.rand.org/pubs/research_reports/RR1165z2.html

Institute of Medicine, *Crossing the Quality Chasm: A New Health System for the 21st Century*, Washington, D.C.: National Academies Press, 2001.

King, Paul R., Kerry T. Donnelly, James P. Donnelly, Mina Dunnam, Gary Warner, C. J. Kittleson, Charles B. Bradshaw, Michelle Alt, and Scott T. Meier, "Psychometric Study of the Neurobehavioral Symptom Inventory," *Journal of Rehabilitation Research and Development*, Vol. 49, No. 6, 2012, pp. 879–888.

Kroenke, Kurt, Robert L. Spitzer, and Janet B. Williams, "The PHQ-9: Validity of a Brief Depression Severity Measure," *General Internal Medicine*, Vol. 9, September 2001, pp. 606–613.

Mattox, Teryn, Kimberly A. Hepner, Daniel R. Kivlahan, Carrie M. Farmer, Susan Rosenbluth, Katherine Hoggatt, Shauna Stahlman, David De Vries, Sean Grant, Harold Alan Pincus, and Katherine E. Watkins, *Candidate Quality Measures to Assess Care for Alcohol Misuse: Technical Specifications*, Santa Monica, Calif.: RAND Corporation, TL-197-NIAAA, 2016. As of December 3, 2021:
https://www.rand.org/pubs/tools/TL197.html

McLellan, A. Thomas, "Substance Misuse and Substance Use Disorders: Why Do They Matter in Healthcare?" *Transactions of the American Clinical and Climatological Association*, Vol. 128, 2017, pp. 112–130.

Minkoff, Kenneth, "Best Practices: Developing Standards of Care for Individuals with Co-Ocurring Psychiatric and Substance Use Disorders," *Psychiatric Services*, Vol. 52, No. 5, pp. 597–599.

Mott, Juliette M., Natalie E. Hundt, Shubhada Sansgiry, Joseph Mignogna, and Jeffrey A. Cully, "Changes in Psychotherapy Utilization Among Veterans with Depression, Anxiety, and PTSD," *Psychiatric Services*, Vol. 65, No. 1, January 1, 2014, pp. 106–112.

Moyer, Virginia A., "Screening and Behavioral Counseling Interventions in Primary Care to Reduce Alcohol Misuse: U.S. Preventive Services Task Force Recommendation Statement," *Annals of Internal Medicine*, August 6, 2013.

National Committee for Quality Assurance, "Initiation and Engagement of Alcohol and Other Drug Abuse or Dependence Treatment (IET)," webpage, 2021a. As of December 3, 2021:
https://www.ncqa.org/hedis/measures/initiation-and-engagement-of-alcohol-and-other-drug-abuse-or-dependence-treatment/

National Committee for Quality Assurance, "HEDIS Measures and Technical Resources," webpage, 2021b. As of December 3, 2021:
https://www.ncqa.org/hedis/measures/

National Quality Forum, "Measures, Reports & Tools," webpage, 2021. As of December 3, 2021:
https://www.qualityforum.org/Measures_Reports_Tools.aspx

NCQA—*See* National Committee for Quality Assurance.

NQF—*See* National Quality Forum.

Penchansky, Roy, and J. William Thomas, "The Concept of Access: Definition and Relationship to Consumer Satisfaction," *Medical Care*, Vol. 19, No. 2, 1981.

Puetz, Timothy W., Shawn D. Youngstedt, and Matthew P. Herring, "Effects of Pharmacotherapy on Combat-Related PTSD, Anxiety, and Depression: A Systematic Review and Meta-Regression Analysis," *PLoS One*, Vol. 10, No. 5, May 2015.

Schlosser, James, Donald Kollisch, Deborah Johnson, Troi Perkins, and Ardis Olson, "VA-Community Dual Care: Veteran and Clinician Perspectives," *Journal of Community Health*, Vol. 45, No. 4, August 2020, pp. 795–802.

Smucker, Sierra, Eric R. Pedersen, and Terri Tanielian, *Improving Behavioral Health Care Access and Treatment Options for Veterans with Co-Occurring Behavioral Health Problems*, Santa Monica, Calif.: RAND Corporation, WR-1328-MTF, 2019. As of December 3, 2021:
https://www.rand.org/pubs/working_papers/WR1328.html

Substance Abuse and Mental Health Services Administration, *Treating Clients with Traumatic Brain Injury (Updated)*, North Bethesday, Md., August 2021. As of December 3, 2021:
https://store.samhsa.gov/sites/default/files/SAMHSA_Digital_Download/PEP21-05-03-001.pdf

Tanielian, Terri, Carrie M. Farmer, Rachel M. Burns, Erin Lindsey Duffy, and Claude Messan Setodji, *Ready or Not? Assessing the Capacity of New York State Health Care Providers to Meet the Needs of Veterans*, Santa Monica, Calif.: RAND Corporation, RR-2298-NYSHF, 2018. As of December 3, 2021:
https://www.rand.org/pubs/research_reports/RR2298.html

Tanielian, Terri, and Lisa H. Jaycox, *Invisible Wounds of War: Psychological and Cognitive Injuries, Their Consequences, and Services to Assist Recovery*, Santa Monica, Calif.: RAND Corporation, MG-720-CCF, 2008. As of December 3, 2021:
https://www.rand.org/pubs/monographs/MG720.html

Teeters, Jenni B., Cynthia L. Lancaster, Delisa G. Brown, and Sudie E. Back, "Substance Use Disorders in Military Veterans: Prevalence and Treatment Challenges," *Substance Abuse and Rehabilitation*, Vol. 8, 2017, pp. 69–77.

Trivedi, Ranak B., Edward P. Post, Haili Sun, Andrew Pomerantz, Andrew J. Saxon, John D. Piette, Charles Maynard, Bruce Arnow, Idamay Curtis, Stephan D. Fihn, and Karin Nelson, "Prevalence, Comorbidity, and Prognosis of Mental Health Among US Veterans," *American Journal of Public Health*, Vol. 105, No. 12, 2015, pp. 2564–2569.

U.S. Department of Veterans Affairs, *VA/DoD Clinical Practice Guidelines: Management of Depressive Disorder (MDD)*, Washington, D.C., 2016. As of December 3, 2021:
https://www.healthquality.va.gov/guidelines/MH/mdd/

U.S. Department of Veterans Affairs, *VA/DoD Clinical Practice Guidelines: Management of Posttraumatic Stress Disorder and Acute Stress Reaction 2017*, Washington, D.C., 2017. As of December 3, 2021:
https://www.healthquality.va.gov/guidelines/MH/ptsd/

U.S. Department of Veterans Affairs, *VA/DoD Clinical Practice Guidelines: The Assessment and Management of Patients at Risk for Suicide*, Washington, D.C., 2019. As of December 3, 2021:
https://www.healthquality.va.gov/guidelines/MH/srb/
VADoDSuicideRiskCPGProviderSummaryFinal5088212019.pdf

U.S. Department of Veterans Affairs, *VA/DoD Clinical Practice Guidelines: Management of Substance Use Disorders (SUD)*, Washington, D.C., 2021a. As of December 3, 2021:
https://www.healthquality.va.gov/guidelines/mh/sud/index.asp

U.S. Department of Veterans Affairs, "MISSION Act Quality Standards," webpage, 2021b. As of December 3, 2021:
https://www.accesstocare.va.gov/Healthcare/MissionActQualityStandards

U.S. Department of Veterans Affairs, *VA/DoD Clinical Practice Guidelines: Management and Rehabilitation of Post-Acute Mild Traumatic Injury (mTBI)*, 2021c. As of December 3, 2021:
https://www.healthquality.va.gov/guidelines/Rehab/mtbi/

VA—*See* U.S. Department of Veterans Affairs.

VHA TRAIN, "Welcome to VHA TRAIN," homepage, undated. As of December 3, 2021:
https://www.train.org/vha/welcome

Weathers, F. W., B. T. Litz, T. M. Keane, P. A. Palmieri, B. P. Marx, and P. P. Schnurr, "The PTSD Checklist for *DSM-5* (PCL-5)," scale available from the National Center for PTSD, 2013. As of September 20, 2021:
https://www.ptsd.va.gov/professional/assessment/adult-sr/ptsd-checklist.asp